Enzyme Power

Tracy K. Gibbs, PhD

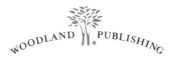

WOODLAND PUBLISHING

For permissions, ordering information, or bulk quantity discounts, contact:
Woodland Publishing, Inc., Salt Lake City, UT

Visit our Web site: www.woodlandpublishing.com
Toll-free number: (800) 777-BOOK (2665)

The information in this book is for educational purposes only and is not recommended as a means of diagnosing or treating an illness. All matters concerning physical and mental health should be supervised by a health practitioner knowledgeable in treating that particular condition. Neither the publisher nor the author directly or indirectly dispenses medical advice, nor do they prescribe any remedies or assume any responsibility for those who choose to treat themselves.

Cataloging-in-Publication data is available from the Library of Congress.

ISBN 978-1-58054-482-5

Printed in the United States of America

Contents

Enzyme Power 5

What Are Enzymes? 5

Different Types of Enzymes 6

What Do Enzymes *Do*? 7

Our Enzyme Bank 7

Maximizing Your Enzyme Levels 8

How Are Enzymes Depleted? 9

Enzyme Activators 11

Dr. Pottenger's Cats 12

Medical Digestion Dilemma 14

Malabsorption Due to Enzyme Deficiency 15

Your Blood Speaks! 16

Does a Lack of Enzymes Contribute to Obesity? 17

Enzymes and Weight Loss 18

Overweight and Sick Children 19

Sugar 20

Osteoporosis 20

Candidiasis and Allergy Relief 21

Will Food Alone Help? 22

So What Should I Do? 22

Good Water Is Also Essential 23

The Enzyme Stomach 23

Plant-based Enzyme Supplements 25

The Power of the Enzyme 26

References 27

Enzyme Power

While many people have heard about enzymes, it's likely that most don't understand the myriad functions they perform in the human body. Enzymes are as critical to life as air and water for all living creatures, including humans. Enzymes make life itself possible—they are the reason why we have energy, why we can reproduce, why we can think, and why we can grow and heal. Enzymes are the building blocks and the life-force of all living things. Simply put, in a world without enzymes, seeds wouldn't sprout, fruit wouldn't ripen, leaves wouldn't change color, living things wouldn't reproduce, and you, as a human being, would not exist.

Enzymes are involved in all of our body systems, including building body mass, detoxifying major organs, and healing injured tissues. Enzymes allow our bodies to digest, absorb, and convert food into energy. They also regulate thousands of other biochemical functions, including respiration, thought, growth, smell, taste, nerve stimulation, immunity, hormone regulation, cellular growth, and the repair of organs, glands, and tissues.

What Are Enzymes?

Enzymes are composed of long chains of amino acids held together by peptide bonds. But this isn't a complete answer, because there's much more to an enzyme than a simple protein. In fact, it is theorized that amino acids only serve as carriers for vital enzyme activity factors—much like a driver in a car. Together they are one, but in fact, they are two separate things. Debate rages as to whether enzymes are types of amino acids or proteins or if they're just "drivers" on amino acid chains. A lot of evidence suggests that enzymes are much more than simple proteins, but a full explanation of this is beyond the scope of this book. Our focus will be on the vital work that enzymes perform within our bodies and ways that we can maximize our enzyme levels.

Different Types of Enzymes

Basically, there are two sources, or classifications, of enzymes:

1. **Endogenous:** originating within the body

2. **Exogenous:** originating outside the body

Within these two sources, there are three distinct classifications of enzymes:

1. **Metabolic enzymes:** work in the blood, tissues, and organs

2. **Digestive enzymes:** help the body convert foods into usable nutrients; secreted by the liver and pancreas

3. **Food enzymes** (found in all raw, unprocessed food): contain digestive enzymes that help break down nutrients during digestion and assist in plant decomposition

Enzymes exist *only* in organic living matter. You cannot obtain or produce enzymes from something that has no life, which means that you cannot get enzymes from minerals, processed foods, or synthetic chemicals.

What Do Enzymes *Do*?

Enzymes are the workforce of the body. A good analogy is to liken enzymes to a construction crew working inside you. This crew uses various raw materials, such as amino acids, fatty acids, sugars, and hormones to build the entire infrastructure the body needs to perform efficiently. This process continues throughout our lives—as long as nutrients are provided in abundance. Without the proper raw materials, enzymes can do nothing. For this reason, vitamin and mineral deficiencies can have devastating effects on the body, so an adequate intake of nutrients is critical. An interesting catch-22 is that—without enzymes—your body will not benefit as it should from getting an adequate supply of vitamins and minerals. Thus, we see that a great circle of nutrients must be consumed to maintain optimal health and that supplementing or eating just a few of these nutrients will serve little, if any, purpose—*especially if we lack abundant enzymes*! Finally, to complete our construction-crew analogy, enzymes also act as a demolition team that cleans up worn-out parts and destroys harmful materials that prevent health and growth.

Our Enzyme Bank

Enzyme deficiency, or exhaustion of the body's enzyme production, leads to aging, disease, and death. According to Dr. Edward Howell, author of *Enzyme Nutrition: The Food Enzyme Concept*, enzyme shortages are commonly seen in patients suffering from chronic illnesses, such as certain types of cancer, allergies, aging, skin disorders, obesity and heart disease. Researchers have proven that the root cause of most disease in humans and domesticated animals stems from nutritional deficiencies. Many researchers are also convinced that virtually all disease may be traced to missing enzymes or malfunctioning enzyme reactions. Without enzymes, the body cannot function properly, nor can essential nutrients be delivered to the cells where they are needed. Dr. Howell likens our bodies to an "enzyme bank." Through our raw food intake we can generally maintain a large number of enzymes in our bodies, like depositing funds into a bank every time we eat raw enzyme-rich food. But once the enzymes are depleted (withdrawn), there are no loans on enzymes, only enzyme bankruptcy, which leads to the slow, degenerative condition of disease.

Generally, low enzyme levels have been associated with older people and people suffering from chronic degenerative diseases, whereas high enzyme levels are usually found in infants and those who are young and healthy. However, anyone can become enzyme deficient at any age if their diet and lifestyle choices are poor. Typically a twenty-year-old will have twice the enzyme level of a seventy-year-old. A newborn baby will have one hundred times more enzymes in her bloodstream than an elderly person. Research has shown that elderly people can maintain high blood enzyme levels simply by consuming a diet high in enzyme-rich foods, such as fermented foods and raw foods, as well as enzyme supplements.

Maximizing Your Enzyme Levels

Your immunity, vitality, and longevity depend on keeping your body's enzyme production at optimal levels. Many factors can help us to maximize our enzyme levels. Genetics—including the health of our parents before and after conception—play a large role in having healthy enzyme levels. However, there are many other factors that have nothing to do with genetics and everything to do with our own eating habits.

Most people are born with the innate ability to manufacture adequate enzymes to maintain good health, and as the years pass, depending on our diets and environment, we can maintain healthy enzyme activity into old age. But if we fail to supply our bodies with the raw materials needed to manufacture these enzymes, over a period of time our bodies will slowly become enzyme deficient. The results of this will be a shorter life.

Your body is like a factory, and its finished product is your energy. In order for us to enjoy an energetic, long, and healthy life, we must avoid metabolic enzyme depletion by providing optimal raw materials for enzyme production. The optimal materials our bodies need to produce our life energy are nutrient-dense, enzyme-rich foods. Our bodies need exogenous food enzymes to help break down food during the digestive process into nutrients that can be assimilated. You might be wondering why—if our bodies already produce digestive enzymes—do we need food enzymes. As a factory, the body continually needs raw materials to produce its finished product. If the body is continually overburdened by having to manufacture energy with only the raw materials it produces, it will begin to break down and wear out. By ingesting exogenous enzymes, we restore our body's raw material supply, like bringing on a temporary crew, thus allowing the body's main crew to rest. If your main crew fails to rest, it doesn't matter what age you are, the stage is set for accelerated aging and disease. Dr. Francis Pottenger discovered this when he conducted studies on several generations of cats with induced enzyme deficiencies. We'll talk about this experiment a little more later on.

There are several well-documented cases of cultures in which many people live in excellent health for over a hundred years. Scientists can keep cells alive and healthy in the laboratory indefinitely. Our bodies have the same potential for longevity, so why are so many people getting sick and dying early? The answer is simple: We eat dead food, food that has been processed beyond our body's ability to recognize it as a nutrient. We add enzyme inhibitors (preservatives) to our food that sap our own body's supply of enzymes as well. We live in a country of abundance, yet astonishingly, many Americans are enzyme deficient and face nutritional bankruptcy. This disaster is not only a problem in the United States, but worldwide. Why?

How Are Enzymes Depleted?

The most serious threat to the body's supply of endogenous enzymes is the habit of eating only cooked and processed foods. Cooking or processing food over 118 degrees Fahrenheit (56 degrees Celsius) completely destroys any enzymes in the food. This means that foods found in a box, a bottle, or a can are dead foods that cannot restore our supply of enzymes. Overcooking of raw organic food also contributes to nutrient loss. Pasteurization, sterilization, radiation, preservation, freezing, and microwaving either render food enzymes inactive or alter their structure so much that they're useless to the body.

Consider all the creatures on the earth. Do you see any form of naturally occurring enzyme depletion within the circle of life's food chain? Human beings and their pets are the only ones that live without food enzymes in their diets.

We just don't see animals in the wild suffering from heart disease, indigestion, acid reflux, diabetes, chronic fatigue, arthritis, and other common lifestyle diseases. But we do see our pets suffering from these diseases.

Fresh, unprocessed foods supply us with the necessary enzymes and coenzymes required by our bodies to function properly. Unfortunately, most people don't eat enough fresh, whole foods to compensate for the enzyme-deficient foods they do eat. Our diets need to include about 60 percent fresh, raw foods so our bodies can handle the other 40 percent of cooked and processed foods. If everyone actually followed a 60/40 ratio of raw to cooked food, we would see degenerative diseases disappear. This simple truth has been proven in numerous studies.

As a result of this, we have been forced into making a choice to maintain good health: Do I eat a diet comprised of 60 percent raw food, or do I take an enzyme supplement with each meal? Fortunately, food enzyme dietary supplements are available. Medical research shows that food enzyme supplements are helpful during the digestive process. By boosting immunity, they help to prevent and fight illnesses and slow the effects of aging, just as our diet would if 60 percent of it were comprised of raw food.

Hundreds of other factors cause enzyme depletion in our bodies and our foods. All of these are human-made and all can lead to degenerative diseases. Because of chemical poisoning, pollution, and soil exhaustion, our earth no longer can provide us with clean air to breathe, pure water to drink, or nutrient-rich foods to eat. The misuse and demineralization of our soils have escalated to such a degree that if nothing is done, all of our foods will contain nothing but empty calories. This is why many food manufacturers add synthetic vitamins and minerals to breakfast cereals, breads, and other grain products.

People all over the world are facing catastrophic diseases directly related to vitamin and mineral deficiencies. Remember, without vitamins and minerals, enzymes are useless.

Other factors such as stress, overly strenuous exercise, pregnancy, frequent colds, exposure to extreme temperatures, and high fevers all require and use a tremendous amount of enzymes. Fried foods, alcohol, drugs, tobacco, and caffeine and other stimulants also significantly increase the quantities of metabolic enzymes produced by the body, which generates cell-damaging substances called free radicals.

Free radicals are highly reactive, unstable oxygen molecules that destroy healthy cell structures, metabolic enzymes, and other protein molecules. Sunlight, radiation, chemical solvents, and pesticides are more examples of cell-damaging substances that generate free radicals and thus weaken our own metabolic supply of enzymes. Free radicals can interfere with DNA coding so severely that the body may make mutated enzymes that cannot function and cells that cannot reproduce. Some researchers believe this is a major cause of Parkinson's disease and other degenerative nerve disorders.

Our bodies try to protect us from free radical damage by producing an enzyme called superoxide dismutase (SOD), which scavenges and neutralizes free radicals. In addition to being an enzyme, SOD is the most powerful natural antioxidant in the body. The most widely known exogenous protective antioxidants are beta-carotene; vitamins A, C, and E; and selenium and zinc, but SOD is over 2,000 times more powerful at scavenging free radicals when compared to these exogenous antioxidants. Antioxidant enzymes help to improve circulation, reduce inflammation, and bond with collagen to promote cellular integrity and flexibility and create more youthful looking skin.

Enzyme Activators

Though very efficient at what they do, enzymes cannot perform any task or function without first being activated by a coenzyme, or helper. Coenzymes, which come from essential vitamins and minerals, are needed for enzymes to function effectively. Enzymes are usually activated by electrical charges contained in trace and macro minerals. Vitamins are usually riders on the enzyme that "drive" the enzyme to a specific function. Imagine that an enzyme is a light bulb. If you purchased a light bulb from your local hardware store, what function could you perform with that light bulb if you didn't first screw it into a socket and turn on the power switch? An enzyme can only function with the electrical charge of the mineral, and the direction or "light switch" of the vitamin. Therefore, all three are necessary to maintain a healthy body.

Each enzyme has a very specific function to perform in the body. This function is determined by the arrangement of amino acids and the distribution of energy each enzyme contains. The basic functioning of the nervous system is one example of the critical role electrical energy plays in our body. The nervous system uses electrical energy via nerve impulses to transmit messages from one cell in the body to another. Muscle movement, glandular secretion, temperature regulation, and even our thought processes depend on electrical energy. This vital energy is considered the life-force of enzymes and cannot be synthetically reproduced.

Enzymes initiate, accelerate, and terminate critical metabolic processes by catalytic action. A catalyst is a substance that can initiate a chemical reaction. Sometimes a catalyst is used up during an activation process and sometimes it is not. Such is the case with enzymes. Specific enzymes bond with molecules and perform chemical reactions such as synthesizing, joining, dividing, and duplicating the molecules. For example, some enzymes break down large nutrients into smaller molecules for digestion and assimilation. Other enzymes are responsible for functions such as respiration, reproduction, vision, and the release and storage of energy. When the reaction is complete, some enzymes are ready to start another reaction, while others will need to be replaced with a new supply to start the process again.

Dr. Pottenger's Cats

Dr. Francis M. Pottenger Jr. (1901–67) has received wide acclaim for a clinical study he conducted to determine the long-term effects of eating cooked foods. The study involved pairing two sets of cats (one male and one female in each pair) and tracking their health over the course of ten years. During the study, Dr. Pottenger fed the two sets of cats raw milk and raw meat, and he fed another three sets of cats pasteurized milk and cooked meat. By the second generation, the cats that ate raw food were, on average, stronger in muscle and bone mass, healthy, and free of disease. They produced healthy kittens generation after generation. At the end of the second generation, the cooked-food-fed cats were weaker in bone structure, mentally slower, and began to suffer from allergies, infections, and other maladies, including kidney, heart, thyroid, and gum diseases. Each succeeding generation of cooked-food cats showed progressively more illness and disease. Over 30 percent of the third generation of cooked-food cats could not produce offspring.

If we compare ourselves to the cats in Dr. Pottenger's study, it's interesting to note that we are now into the third generation of humans to eat predominantly cooked and processed foods. Our grandparents began eating this way after World War I, when canned foods became common and food processing became a financial necessity for mass production and distribution of food.

Are you wondering what I'm wondering here? If 30 percent of Dr. Pottenger's cats couldn't reproduce after three generations of eating cooked food, where will *we* be after three, four, or five generations? Recent studies reveal that men's sperm counts have plummeted over the last two generations. No one yet knows if there's a direct correlation with diet, but this development is certainly cause for concern.

Whether we are cats, dogs, or human beings, when we eat enzyme-deficient food, our bodies are overburdened by the need to produce enzymes to help process what we eat. The body will actually interrupt the production of vital metabolic enzymes to compensate for the enzyme deficiencies in the foods we eat. Several theories claim that the human body is only capable of producing a certain amount of metabolic enzymes. When this supply is gone, your body will stop functioning and you will die. Edward Howell said this in 1930, and now thousands of doctors are beginning to agree. Only by ingesting food enzymes can we stop our bodies from being depleted of the nutrients that are essential for a healthy life.

Medical Digestion Dilemma

Signs of enzyme deficiency are all around us, and each comes with its own set of symptoms, including heartburn, gas, bloating, and acid reflux. Other symptoms include headaches, chronic fatigue, stomachaches, diarrhea, constipation, yeast infections, and a variety of nutritional deficiencies. Because these symptoms are so common today, many people think they're normal. But they're not normal—they're a plain indication that our bodies can no longer process the food that modern agriculture and food processors produce for us. These dead foods will affect all of our digestive organs, namely the stomach, intestines, colon, liver, pancreas, and gall bladder. We know there's a problem out there: Over-the-counter sales for Tums and Rolaids antacids topped $3.8 billion in the United States in 2002.

Could supplementing our diets with enzymes or eating more raw food save our country billions of dollars in health-care costs? Digestive disease is the most common reason for hospitalization—more than any other disease category. Americans spend more than $50 billion a year for surgical procedures and other treatments related to digestive diseases. Digestive complaints are the major reason given for absenteeism from work and school. Eating enzyme-less food compromises every aspect of the digestive process: digestion, absorption, assimilation, and elimination. All of these processes are essential for good nutrition and a healthy body.

Autopsies have shown that people who primarily eat cooked foods have a dangerously enlarged and poorly functioning pancreas. If the pancreas is stressed day after day, year after year, in order to produce an excess of digestive enzymes, then the rest of the body's enzyme reserve is severely taxed. Most young people appear to suffer no ill effects from this overtaxing. But appearances are frequently deceiving. Gradually, the overworked pancreas and other digestive organs will not be able to produce sufficient quantities of endogenous metabolic enzymes. This leads to digestive diseases and a toxic bowel condition. According to Edward Howell in *Enzyme Nutrition,* an enlarged pancreas is correlated to an increased incidence of chronic degenerative diseases and cancer. He also showed that an adult human's pancreas that had a digestive disease was the same size as an adult healthy cow's pancreas, even though the cow had five times the diseased individual's body mass. This, he said, "was proof that the body will continue to enlarge the pancreas so as to secrete more digestive enzymes, thus taxing the other organs of the body and causing death."

Malabsorption Due to Enzyme Deficiency

Sadly we know that today's typical diet seriously lacks enzymes, but our typical diet also lacks another essential element—fiber. Fiber acts as a bulking agent and speeds transit time of food through the digestive tract. These actions prevent metabolic waste from creating toxic by-products. A major benefit of fiber is that it binds acids to bile and carries the bile along with excess fats out of the body. Fiber helps to lower cholesterol, reduce the risk of heart disease, lower blood pressure, improve blood sugar levels, and promote the growth of friendly intestinal flora. It also promotes bowel regularity, aids digestion by giving the digestive enzymes more time to work, and helps promote overall bowel health.

Fiber cannot do its job effectively unless enzymes do theirs. Over time, hard-to-digest high-protein foods (such as cooked meat and other enzyme-deficient foods) exhaust the digestive organs until they can no longer function efficiently. This results in the accumulation of partially digested food in the bowel. By middle age, many people have pounds of undigested, putrefactive food in their colon. Toxins produced from this buildup are reabsorbed into the bloodstream, creating autointoxication, or self-poisoning. This results in a dramatically weakened immune system and can lead to seriously debilitating health conditions, including colon cancer, the most common form of cancer in the United States. Eating more raw enzyme-rich foods and/or taking supplemental food enzymes with meals and between meals can help eliminate the accumulation of toxic wastes.

Your Blood Speaks!

Live blood cell morphology is the science behind the size and shape or pattern of red blood cells in the body. This informative science can help identify many nutritional deficiencies before they become diagnosable diseases. I began teaching live blood cell morphology classes in 1995 and have found it to be a very effective tool. Some traditional medical doctors may question its usefulness because their training emphasizes diagnosing disease, and live blood cell morphology doesn't do that. But it can be quite helpful in other ways

Both traditional medical doctors and homeopathic practitioners use live blood cell morphology to prescreen individuals to determine if they need further tests. By examining a patient's blood through a microscope, the practitioner can see excess proteins, fats, and sugars in the bloodstream that can lead to a myriad of health problems. Excess protein will create uric acid and contribute to the deterioration of muscle and joints. Excess fats such as triglycerides can clog major arteries and cause heart attacks and strokes. Certain types of enzymes can act as scavengers to eliminate excess food residues in our bloodstream. When we consume foods that are high in proteins, fats, and sugars yet lack these live enzymes to process the nutrients, our immune system can become overworked because it's forced to "clean up" after our meals. This process could lead to numerous diseases, including allergies, rheumatoid arthritis, and cancer, among others.

During illness and infection, white blood cell production increases to fight off pathogens. When we overeat cooked foods, our bodies react as if we had an acute illness. Within thirty minutes of eating cooked foods, our white blood cell count increases dramatically. This means the immune system is being unnecessarily called into action virtually every time we eat.

Studies show that the increased production and mobilization of white blood cells do not occur when only raw food is consumed. Molecules from improperly digested proteins and fats that are small enough to get into the blood, but too large to get into the cells, are called floating immune complexes. They are now considered toxic invaders in the body instead of nutrients.

A microscope used for live blood cell analysis is an excellent tool to show a patient how these excess nutrients in the bloodstream can negatively affect their health. A typical research-grade microscope can magnify a tiny drop of blood 1,000 times, and by projecting that on a TV monitor you can actually see a red blood cell that's twenty thousand times its actual size. By doing this, you can view an accurate real-time picture of your blood cells.

Under a microscope we can see what happens to red blood cells when proteins are not properly assimilated or digested. This causes the red blood cells to stick together, which results in a lack of surface area and creates low oxygen content and poor nutrient delivery. This condition would lead to chronic fatigue, migraine headaches, stiff muscles and poor circulation. We could also see the effects of long-term protein consumption manifest as digestive problems such as the formation of uric acid crystals, which could eventually lead to arthritis and gout. Using a microscope we can also see chylos (undigested fats from your last meal) and plaque, which can lead to arteriosclerosis. It takes a concentrated effort on the part of our white blood cells to eliminate these excess foods and protect our bodies from other toxic invaders. If raw food is not consumed and digested properly on a regular basis, you can clearly see the many health problems that such an unhealthy habit can cause.

Does a Lack of Enzymes Contribute to Obesity?

Who needs research to see that over 120 million Americans are now overweight? I travel abroad extensively and all I have to do is fly back to the United States and look around to realize the difference in the size of the average American versus the average European or Asian. It reminds me of the paintings of corpulent Romans reclining on their plush sofas oblivious to the fact that lean, fit Germanic tribes were about to invade their borders to the north. So too will disease and other degenerative conditions invade America's lifestyle of excess if we don't begin to take action. The average person's diet today consists of too many processed and cooked foods that are high in empty calories, processed sugars, and trans fats. Our typical diet is also low in fiber and essential enzymes. Excess body fat, caused by empty calorie intake and lack of exercise, is associated with many diseases. Additionally, virtually all health studies agree that excess body fat can significantly shorten your life span.

Many Americans believe that fat from food is bad for you, but fat from both plants and animals is one of the best sources of energy available—as long as it's in its original, unprocessed form. For example, in the not-so-distant past, the Eskimo diet consisted mainly of uncooked animal protein and whale blubber. Generations of Eskimos lived on this diet without suffering from nutritional deficiencies. In fact, they were extremely robust and healthy and were not afflicted with conditions such as high blood pressure, high cholesterol, heart disease, kidney stones, or other modern lifestyle diseases.

The Masai tribes in Africa are much the same way. They sustained themselves on a diet of beef fat and milk in its raw form. Again, after hundreds of autopsies, no heart disease and no clogged arteries were found. Today, things are very different. Most Eskimos and most Masai have adopted the Western practice of eating cooked and processed food and have now inherited the degenerative diseases associated with an enzyme-less diet. It is the enzymes in the unprocessed foods that kept them healthy for generations, and it is the enzyme-less diets that are now causing them to inherit our human-made diseases.

Enzymes and Weight Loss

One of the primary keys to weight loss may simply be the action of enzymes. Dr. David Galton at Tufts University School of Medicine tested people weighing 230–240 pounds. He found that virtually all of them were lacking lipase enzymes in their fatty tissues. Lipase, which is found abundantly in raw foods, is a fat-splitting enzyme that aids the body in digestion, the storage and distribution of fat, and the burning of fat for energy. Lipase activity breaks down and dissolves fat throughout the body. Without lipase, fat stagnates and accumulates in the organs, arteries, and capillaries.

A good example of the importance of lipase activity lies in an interesting experiment with pigs. Veterinarians fed one group of pigs only enzyme-rich raw potatoes and another group enzyme-deficient cooked potatoes. The pigs that ate the raw potatoes did not get fat. However, the pigs that ate the cooked potatoes gained weight rapidly. The regular use of digestive food enzymes that include lipase with meals often results in shedding excess pounds.

Overweight and Sick Children

Before the advent of processed foods, junk foods, and fast foods, overweight children were rare, and because they were rare, they were deemed to be healthy and typically represented high social status and wealth. Recently, I spent a day with my darling nieces and was astounded by how much processed food they consumed in less than four hours—the three of them together finished off an entire *pound* of sugar! They are also, unfortunately, overweight for their ages and will suffer for their choices if they don't change what they eat.

A simple experiment can help you clearly see what's happening to kids today. Go to any shopping mall and you'll see overweight children and teenagers that are part of our epidemic of obesity and overweight, an epidemic that will cost society trillions of dollars in health-care costs, not to mention the tragic human toll in suffering, death, and loss. According to 1998 statistics, a minimum of 25 percent of U.S. children were overweight. This is an increase of 33 percent since 1978 studies. A 2002 study of a local school system indicated that 34 percent of children were overweight. That's a 10 percent increase in just four years!

Not only are many of our children overweight, but doctors are now treating children for juvenile arthritis, type 2 diabetes, and other degenerative diseases that just a few years ago were found only in people in their fifties and sixties. This disturbing trend is directly related to diets that are high in fats and sugars and low in fiber, enzymes, vitamins, and minerals. According to statistics, less than 1 percent of our children eat the minimum recommended servings of fruits and vegetables on a daily basis. It is not known what percentage of that may be raw. Children can certainly benefit from food enzyme and other nutritional supplements. Children with high enzyme levels will have high energy levels. It's hard to believe that all this could be solved by simply eating more raw food and/or taking a simple capsule with each meal. But it can.

Sugar

What about sugar? Unprocessed raw sugar contains enzymes, chromium, and B vitamins, plus it's easily digested and assimilated. White processed sugar contains no enzymes, no B vitamins, and no chromium. In order for the body to metabolize processed sugar, the missing enzymes, vitamins, and chromium must be stolen from the body's own tissue stores. If large quantities of white sugar are eaten, then not only are the body's enzymes depleted, but we also suffer B-vitamin and chromium deficiencies. Chromium is an essential mineral needed by the body to support efficient insulin function. Insulin regulates the metabolism of proteins, carbohydrates, and fats. Studies show a relationship between obesity, diabetes, and chromium deficiencies. B vitamins are considered coenzymes essential to the metabolism of all cells. Without them, we will continue to raise obese, diabetes-prone children.

Osteoporosis

Calcium is an abundant mineral found in many plants and raw dairy foods. However, without enzymes in the foods, your body cannot fully assimilate the calcium they contain. People diagnosed with osteoporosis are generally told to take calcium and vitamin D supplements. Yet in a few months or years they find that not only has the disorder progressed, but they now have a buildup of calcium in the joints, including bone spurs or blocked arteries due to calcium deposits. Without proper assimilation of calcium from the foods we consume, the body will get its calcium from its bones and muscles. This results in weak, brittle bones and muscular fatigue and cramping.

I am convinced that enzyme supplements are the answer to proper calcium assimilation from the foods we eat and the supplements we take. It is now known that certain types of calcium act as cofactors for enzyme activation of protease. Protease is the enzyme that breaks down and digests proteins, like those found in meat and dairy products.

Isn't it interesting to learn that nature knew we needed the calcium in milk and included exactly the right enzyme in the milk to help us digest it? And what did we do? We started to heat (pasteurize) the milk to kill bacteria, and in the process we've been killing the enzymes as well, thus preventing our bodies from digesting the milk properly, which also prevents our bodies from absorbing the calcium that we needed from the milk in the first place. Does any of this make sense to you?

Candidiasis and Allergy Relief

Candidiasis is an overgrowth of the common yeast *Candida albicans,* which lives in the intestinal tract. The condition typically affects the endocrine and nervous systems and can have a devastating effect on the immune system. Yeast overgrowth can be triggered by several factors. Taking antibiotics regularly will kill the good bacteria in your colon that keep the yeast at bay, thus allowing the yeast to proliferate. Another cause is the large consumption of processed carbohydrates and simple sugars. Yeast spores will feed off of these sugars thus inducing their proliferation. It is estimated that at least 50 percent of the population may be affected by yeast overgrowth, which can lead to allergies of various types, chronic fatigue, and many outward symptoms, such as athlete's foot, jock itch, vaginal and anal yeast infections, and other skin irritations.

Candidiasis and allergies affect millions of people. Allergens and antigens such as viruses, bacteria, fungi, and yeast are most often proteins. They enter the body through the digestive tract. Allergens may also be breathed into the body through the lungs. Protease is a digestive enzyme needed in tremendous quantities to digest and eliminate these toxic invaders, not only in the digestive tract but in the bloodstream as well. Most antigens, including yeast, can be eliminated by taking certain systemic enzyme supplements. Systemic enzymes can be taken both with food at mealtime and in between meals to help digest excess proteins, fats, and sugars in the bloodstream.

Will Food Alone Help?

In today's society, a diet of live organic foods would be almost impossible to attain. Even if we were able to accomplish it, we still may not get our nutritional needs met. Why? Devitalized soil produces devitalized food. Also, our foods are rarely garden fresh, and enzyme loss starts when crops are harvested. Fruits and vegetables contain no enzymes if they aren't allowed to vine ripen. They are often picked green and transported long distances to our supermarkets. Irradiating foods and using other types of preservation to keep food fresh also kills enzymes. Because of deficiencies created over the years from eating cooked food, many people find that even if they do switch to a raw food diet, it doesn't agree with them unless they take enzyme supplements.

So What Should I Do?

Consume as many high-quality raw and freshly juiced fruits and vegetables as possible. They will directly enhance endogenous enzyme activity in your body. Include food enzyme supplements with each meal. I also encourage you to include sprouted superfoods in your diet such as alfalfa and soybeans and green superfoods such as blue-green algae, hydrilla, green barley, chlorella, and spirulina. Superfoods are available in supplement form and contain high-quality predigested proteins, vitamins, antioxidants, minerals, and enzymes.

Trace minerals are needed to activate enzymes, so it's wise to include a full-spectrum mineral supplement to make up for any possible shortages in our diet. Plant-based enzyme supplements taken with both raw and cooked meals can assure optimum digestion and assimilation of the nutrients in the foods we eat. This will relieve stress on the pancreas and allow metabolic enzymes to perform their vital functions throughout the body.

Good Water Is Also Essential

We also need water in our cells, GI tract, and bloodstream to activate enzymes. Water transports oxygen to your body's cells, helps your body to digest and absorb nutrients, and helps eliminate toxins and solid wastes. It lubricates your joints, keeps your skin moist and your organs from sticking together, and maintains proper balance inside and outside your cells. It is critically important to provide your body with the purest water available. Don't drink or cook with water that's been treated with chlorine, a chemical disinfectant that kills harmful bacteria. When ingested, chlorine also kills friendly bacteria in the stomach and colon. For over twenty years, chlorine has been linked to cancers of the colon, rectum, bladder, and prostate.

Our bodies need an adequate supply of pure water every day, and we can meet this need by eating high-water-content foods as well as just drinking water. The amount of water your body needs depends a lot on your environment and your body size. A good average calculation would be to divide your body weight by half and then convert the remainder to ounces. For example, if you weigh 120 pounds, you would need 60 ounces of water a day.

Most people think that as long as they're drinking liquids, they're meeting their body's fluid requirements. Not true. Coffee and alcohol, for example, dehydrate the body and leech essential vitamins and minerals. For the damage done by drinking one cup of coffee or one ounce of alcohol, you will need to drink eight glasses of water to repair your body. In the United States, we spend billions of dollars a year on sodas, coffee, processed juices, and alcoholic beverages—none of which can substitute for your body's basic need for pure water.

The Enzyme Stomach

Digestion actually starts with the nose. The process of smelling food triggers a chemical reaction in the body. Have you ever driven by a fast-food restaurant while you were hungry and the smell alone made your stomach growl and your mouth to salivate? This is due to your good sense of smell. Smelling our food causes the brain to signal for the secretion of salivary amylase and also tells the pancreas and stomach to prepare to ingest food. Through your sense of smell, your body not only recognizes if a food is acidic or alkaline, it also secretes specific enzymes in response to that particular food.

Stage two of the digestion process occurs in the mouth. This is the primary reason why food should be chewed thoroughly before swallowing. Food mixed with the enzyme amylase (produced by the salivary glands) starts predigesting sugars and starches. During the mastication process (chewing), enzymes found naturally in the food also begin the work of predigestion.

Stage three of digestion occurs after the food has been swallowed and then drops down into the upper portion of the stomach. This portion of the stomach is called the cardiac portion or enzyme stomach. The food stays in the enzyme stomach for forty-five minutes to one hour, where natural enzymes or supplemental enzymes continue predigestion of carbohydrates, fats and proteins. It is estimated that enzymes derived from raw food or food-enzyme supplements can actually predigest as much as 75 percent of food in the enzyme stomach without the help of metabolic enzymes secreted by the body.

The fourth stage of digestion occurs in the mid and lower parts of the stomach, where hydrochloric acid and pepsin, chymotrypsin, and several other digestive enzymes made by the body break down the rest of the meal. The final stage of digestion occurs in the duodenum and small intestine, where the pancreas and liver introduce more digestive enzymes to complete digestion. Finally, the converted nutrients pass through the intestinal wall into the bloodstream, ready to be taken by metabolic enzymes throughout the body, to the organs, tissues, nerves, and glands where they're needed.

As you can see, with today's diet and eating habits, stages one, two, and three of the digestive process rarely occur. Why? Because we don't take the time to prepare our food, which allows us to smell it. We don't take the time to properly chew our food, and we don't eat the enzyme-rich foods that are necessary for stage three of the digestive process.

Plant-based Enzyme Supplements

Several varieties of enzyme supplements are available. All digestive enzymes come from a living source, either plant or animal. Pepsin, trypsin, and pancreatin are all derived from animal sources. Since animal-based enzymes work only in very acidic environments, supplements containing them need to be enteric coated. This makes them good for fat digestion and some protein digestion, but they do not work in predigestion or in the blood.

Plant-based enzymes like bromelain, an enzyme produced by pineapples, and papain, an enzyme that comes from the papaya plant, are just the opposite. They work well in the cardiac stomach and assist in the predigestive stages but do nothing for the later stages of digestion as they are rendered inactive at a pH of 4 or lower. They work best at temperatures considerably higher than the body's, which is why in Hawaii they have been traditionally used for slow cooking at low temperatures. Other plant enzymes are good at breaking down mostly plant-based foods. An apple has just enough enzymes in it to digest itself if it was picked when ripe. A cabbage has just enough enzymes in it to break itself down as well, and so forth. So using a plant-based enzyme from multiple plants would allow you to digest a variety of fruits and vegetables, but it wouldn't help much with fatty and protein-rich foods such as meat and dairy products.

Today, the best sources of supplemental enzymes are two species of fungi: *Aspergillus oryzae* and *Aspergillis niger*. They have a much wider range of pH adaptability than animal-derived enzymes and are known to be active in a pH range from 1.7 to 11. In other words, they would work in all stages of digestion, and if you were to take them on an empty stomach, they would even work in your bloodstream. These enzymes come in powders or capsules that can be taken by mouth or sprinkled on food. You will never find these in tablet form because the heat generated by tablet-making machines destroys the aspergillus enzymes, which, like all enzymes are very heat sensitive. For the simple reason that aspergillus-derived enzymes work in all pH levels and can easily be taken orally, I usually recommend that anyone who eats cooked food on a regular basis supplement their diet with them.

When searching for an enzyme supplement, remember that enzymes have very specific functions. For example, the enzyme protease will only digest proteins; amylase digests complex carbohydrates; maltase and sucrase digest complex and simple sugars; lactase digests milk sugars; lipase digests lipids, or fats, and cellulase digests fibers. Make sure you choose a supplement that contains a variety of different enzymes so you won't have to take multiple capsules to digest everything in your meal.

Numerous studies show that people can significantly improve a myriad of medical conditions—such as circulatory and blood pressure problems, hardening of the arteries, arteriosclerosis, diabetes, skin afflictions, and arthritis—by taking supplemental food enzymes. Studies also show that enzyme supplements help with faster recovery time from sports-related injuries. Drs. Lopez, Miehlke, and Williams confirmed the healing properties of enzyme supplementation in their outstanding book *Enzymes: The Foundation of Life,* published by Neville Press in 1994. Unfortunately, the book is out of print, but you may be able to find a copy at your local library or from a used book retailer on the Web. Another good choice is Edward Howell's *Enzyme Nutrition: The Food Enzyme Concept,* which I referred to earlier.

The Power of the Enzyme

To prevent enzyme depletion from shortening your life, you must consume food enzymes in sufficient quantities for your liver and pancreas to adequately digest what you eat. Your body will then be free to produce more metabolic enzymes to help keep you healthy and help prevent the myriad of diseases that plague us today.

References

Adibi, S.A.; Mercer, D.W. "Protein digestion in human intestines as reflected in plasma amino acid concentrations after meals." *J Clin. Invest.* 52 (1973), 1586–594.

Ambrus, J. L. "Absorption of exogenous and endogenous enzymes." *Clinical Pharmacol. Ther.* 8 (1967), 362.

Baintner, K. "Intestinal absorption of enzymes and immune transmission from mother to young." (1986) Boca Raton: CRC.

Boyer P. D., et al. *The Enzymes,* vol. 4. (1960) New York: Academic Press.

Garnder, M. L. G. "Intestinal assimilation of intact peptides and proteins from diet." *Biol. Rev.* 59 (1984), 289–31.

Goldberg, D. M. "Enzymes as agents for the treatment of disease." *Clin. Chimi. Acta* 206 (1992), 45–76.

Heinz, H. P. "Comparison of the effects of 16 different enzymes on serum." *Clinical Immunobiology* 165 (1983), 175–85.

Howell, E. *Enzyme Nutrition: The Food Enzyme Concept.* (1985) New York: Avery Publishing.

Kleine, G. "Enzyme therapy in chronic polyarthritis." *Natural and Holistic Medicine* 1 (1988), 112–16.

Liebow, C. "Enteropancreatic circulation of digestive enzymes." *Science* 189 (1975), 472.

Lopez, D., R. Williams, M. Miehlke. *Enzymes: The Foundation of Life.* (1994) Charleston, SC: Neville Press.

Santillo, H. "Food Enzymes: The Missing Link to Radiant Health. (1987) Prescott, AZ: Holm Press.

Seifert, J. "Qualitative analysis about the absorption of enzymes from the GI tract after oral administration." *General Physician (Allgemeinartz)* 19 (1990): 132.

Steffen, C., J. Manzel, J. Smolen. "Intestinal absorption of an enzyme mixture." *Acta Medica Austriaca* 6 (1979): 13.

Wolf, M., K. Ransberger. *Enzyme Therapy.* (1970) Vienna: Maudrich-Verlag.

About the Author

TRACY K. GIBBS, PHD, attended Aichi Medical School in Aichi, Japan, where he studied hematology, nutrition, pharmacology, advanced herbology, and genetics. In 1995, he received a degree in pharmacology from Kenchi Kenkyu Gakkuin School of Pharmacy in Nagoya, Japan.

Dr. Gibbs has lectured throughout world on the clinical applications of herbal medicine and is the administrator of two schools—one in Japan and one in the United States—that teach heads of households how to use herbs in everyday situations as an alternative to visiting crowded medical clinics.

The author of *Creating Your Own Natural Pharmacy: 33 Do-It-Yourself Herbal Home Remedies* (also published by Woodland), Dr. Gibbs has published two books in Japanese, *Your Blood Speaks* and *Enzyme Power* (titles are translations). He is currently working on completing the first English textbook on performing live cell morphology using methods that have been approved in other countries.